HEALTH
IN A
NUTSHELL
AND
KIDS
HEALTH

LOZZA

Ordering Information:

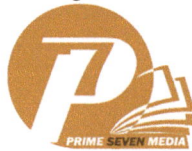

Prime Seven Media
518 Landmann St.
Tomah City, WI 54660

Printed in the United States of America

A healthy low G.I Alternative plus Kids Health

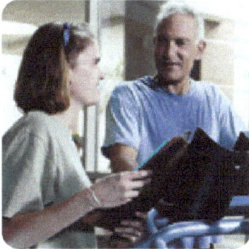

Looking after your health

Keeping your cholesterol low

Easy to do exercises.

Looking after your heart

What is High G.I.

Benefits of low G.I. foods

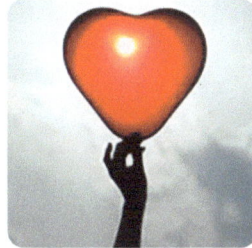

Easy to do recipes for breakfast, Lunch, and dinner.

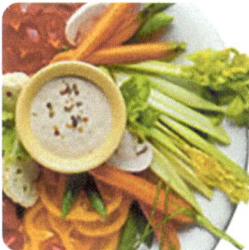

Why do we put on weight?

I can't lose weight.

Tips for eating out.

Plus, much more inside

Healthy eating for Active Kids

Ten ways to get them Active.

Examples of Healthy Snacks

School Lunch Box Ideas

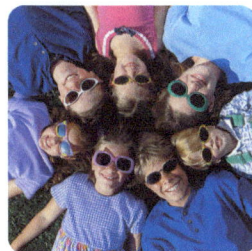

Contents

Carbohydrates are found in many of the Foods we eat each day.

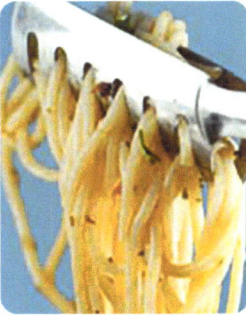

There are a range of different carbohydrates ranging from individual glucose molecules and sugars to larger carbohydrates chains such as starches. Our digestive systems break down carbohydrates to release individual sugar molecules which are absorbed into the bloodstream.

Carbohydrates are essential to maintain blood glucose levels providing fuel to our muscles and brain low blood glucose level (Known as hypoglycemia) can make us feel tired, dizzy, and generally unwell.

Carbohydrate foods are important fuel but also provide an amazing range of vitamins and minerals that are essential for a healthy digestive system.

Not all carbohydrates are digested and absorbed at the same rate and the type of carbohydrate can have a specific influence on health and energy levels.

Sustainability is a major factor, and a healthy food intake should incorporate changes that are long team. Many popular 'diets' are difficult to adhere to and are not enjoyable.

Eating should be pleasurable, and it is important to consume a wide variety of foods for enjoyment and nutritional adequacy.

What is the Glycemic Index?

The Glycemic index (G.I) ranks carbohydrate foods according to their effect on blood glucose levels. High G.I foods are absorbed quickly and can cause a rapid rise in blood glucose levels. Low GI foods are broken down gradually over time and keep blood glucose levels more stable.

Stocking the refrigerator

The grocery store may seem overwhelming when you are trying to eat a low G.I diet. Shopping for food shouldn't be stressful keep the following tips in mind next time you are at the store.

- Don't go shopping hungry; eat a snack to avoid impulse buying.
- Shop the outside edges of the store first, which is where you will usually find the better food choices.
- Check out the ingredients, limit foods with large amounts of sugar, flour, and salt, refined grains, and hydrogenated vegetable oils.
- Peruse the *"NUTRITION FACTS"* look at calorie count, carbohydrate, and fat content for each serving. Also look at the fibre, sodium, and sugar content. Evaluate them against your healthy eating choices and nutrition goals.

☛ Focus on making healthy choices of whole unrefined foods.

☛ Stock up on legumes, whole grain nuts, healthy oils, fruits

☛ Low fat proteins, and light dairy products.

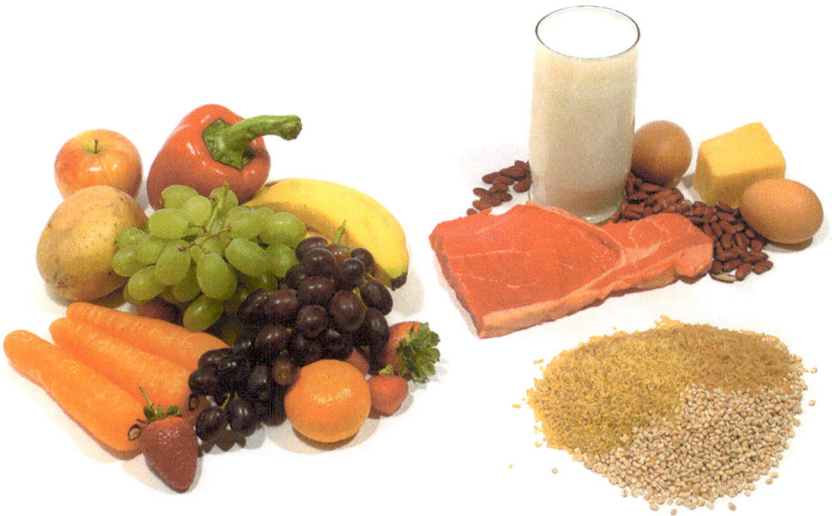

What counts as a serving?

Vegetables
1 cup raw or cooked vegetables
2 cups raw leafy green vegetables
1 large whole pepper
1 large whole tomato

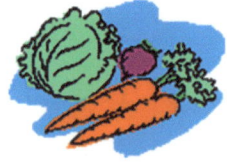

Fruit
1 cup whole fruit juice
1 medium apple or orange
1 cup whole grapes
About 8 large strawberries
1 cup diced melon.

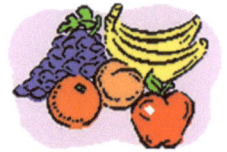

Grain
1 regular slice of bread
1cup of cereal flakes
1/2 English muffin
5 whole wheat crackers
1/2 cup cooked.

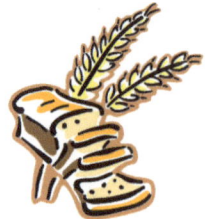

Dairy
1 cup of milk
42g natural cheese

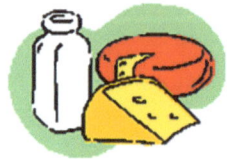

Protein
28g meat, poultry, or fish
1/4 cup cooked dry beans.
1 teaspoon peanut butter
1 egg

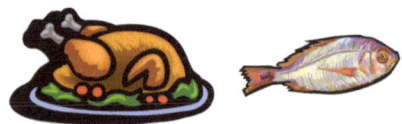

This information will assist in weight control and help realize, *the importance of a low GI diet.* Exercise is a crucial part of the complete program as you make a break from the typical Western diet.

Each day replace your meals and snacks with delicious diet shakes and bars, plus a bonus snack of one *serving of fruit and one serving o vegetables.*

Drink 1-2 liters of water and walk briskly for up to 30 minutes a daily. All the critical components you need for a healthy weight control:

Repair the damage, lose the weight!

Wind back the clock live longer and healthier.

Understand the importance of making good food choices and eat a healthy balanced diet.

The glycogenic index is the key to a lifetime of healthy habits.

It isn't necessary to starve yourself to control weight. In fact, consistently eating less then 1,000 calories a day may actually slow down your

Metabolism and make it harder to control their weight.

You do how ever need to make smarter choices about what you eat.

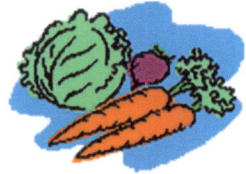

HIGH GI FOODS AND WEIGHT CONTROL

After years of continually abusing their bodies through sedentary habits and eating an improper diet of high GI foods that spike the blood glucose levels many people find it becomes harder and harder to maintain a healthy weight. A poor lifestyle can cause your body to over-stimulate the release of insulin.

The body's storage hormones in essence, if you keep over eating sugar and high GI. Carbohydrates will be more likely to cause you to gain weight.

When you eat high GI foods that are full of fat and sugar, it can cause your body's blood glucose levels to quickly spike and crash, leading to feelings of hunger sooner and craving for more high GI foods.

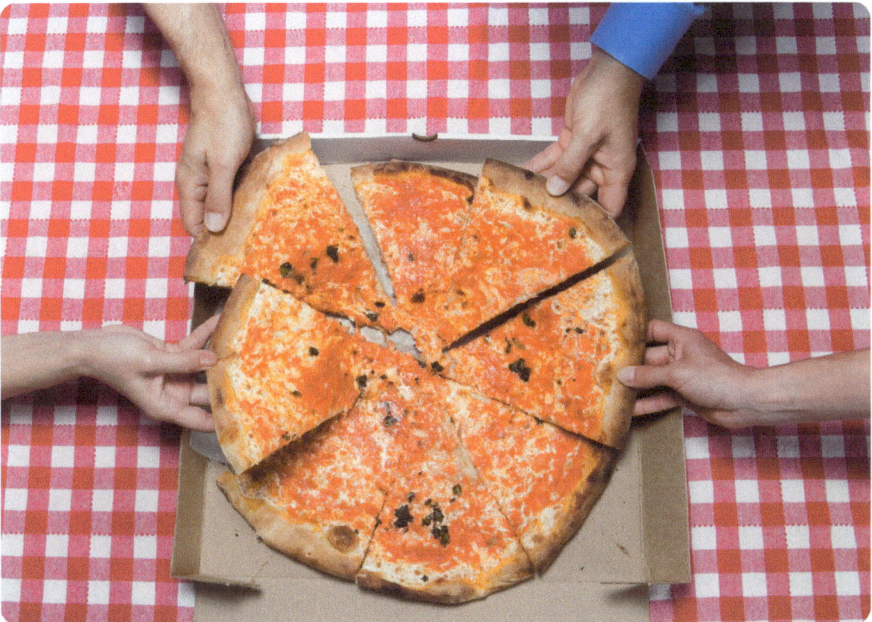

Benefits of Low G.I Foods

1. Stable blood glucose levels resulting in improved energy levels.

2. Reduced cravings for sugar and sweet foods.

3. Keeps you full longer, reducing total daily kilojoules intake.

4. Improved blood glucose control for people with Diabetes.

5. Research shows that a low G.I diet can help to improve blood lipid profile.

6. Active people use a combination of high and low G.I foods to ensure Optimal energy stores for exercise performance.

7. A range of low G.I foods provide important vitamins, minerals and fibre.

It is important to remember that although low G.I carbohydrates are a preferred choice this does not mean you can eat as much as you like.

A mistake many people make is replacing fat in the diet with carbohydrates, often in unlimited and excessive volumes.

Eating too much of any nutrient including carbohydrates can lead to over consumption of kilojoules and this will prevent body fat breakdown and result in subsequent body fat gain. Portion sizes should be appropriate for activity level and individual energy requirements.

A reduction in carbohydrate intake or total calorie intake may be warranted in many situations however severe.

Choose low G.I foods according to how fast they release sugar into the bloodstream (therefore only carbohydrate rich foods Can be classified) low G.I foods release glucose steadily over several hours and therefore less insulin is required leaving you feeling satisfied for longer.

High G.I foods release glucose rapidly increasing the blood sugar levels which turns on fat storage as the body reacts with insulin.

High GI   # low G.I

High GI	low G.I
White bread	Multi grain bread
Rice based crackers	Oats, porridge
muesli	Natural pasta
White rice	Low fat milk or yoghurt
White based breakfast biscuits	Most fruit
glucose	Sweet corn
Jellybeans	Sweet potatoes
White potatoes	legumes
Apple juice	

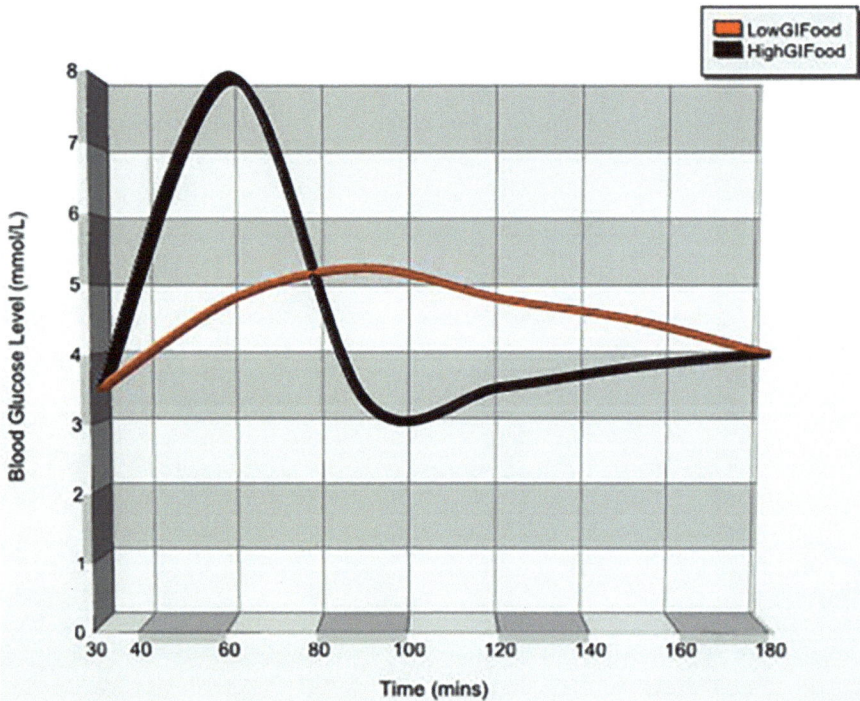

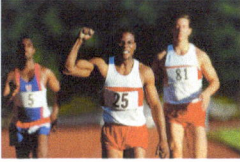

The benefits of walking

Walking can burn fat more than running

Summer is a great time to get into walking one of the easiest and simplest most versatile exercises available today. Walking can produce remarkable results overtime starting slowly and gradually building to a vigorous walk. At least 30mins three or four times a week can improve muscle tone, ease stress, boost your energy level at a moderate for 30 to 60 minutes can build muscle increase your metabolism and burn fat. In fact, you can burn more fat walking then running.

The first step is setting goals, this may sound critical but look at what you want and why. Don't expect too much of yourself in the beginning and become discouraged, also don't start too fast and risk soreness and injury. You must eventually be able to walk 20minutes at a brisk pace without stopping. Don't forget to loosen up, warming up exercises will help alleviate muscle stiffness and pulled muscles. Remember to stretch after you walk to decrease the buildup of lactic acid the chemical, the byproduct that causes muscles to ache.

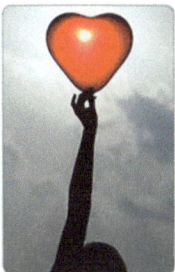

Now it's up to you to make the decision to walk out the door and start down the path to a healthier relaxed you. Take walk it's great! It conditions your heart and lungs and increases the body's ability to use oxygen efficiently.

It acts as a conditioner it conditions your heart and lungs and increases the body's ability to use oxygen efficiently. Everyone knows how to walk, right (not necessarily).

To get the most from your walking walk with your chin up and your shoulders slightly back. Walk so the heel of your foot touches the ground first then roll your weight forward. Swing your arms as you walk for additional exercise. It acts as a protector and helps to reduce the risk of some health problems. It has been shown to reduce the risk of heart attack and stroke and some forms of cancer, and osteoporosis, while taking off fat and building muscle. It's a joint saver walking can burn about as many calories as running but delivers only one quarter of the jolt to your joints and muscles. Most walkers report they feel better, sleep better, and have a much better outlook. Walking has the lowest dropout rate of any form of exercise.

When you finish walking and calculated how many calories you just burned, don't sabotage your efforts to something that will wipe out the gains. It only takes one or two ounces of chips, (about 300 calories) to negate an hour of walking. A snickers bar is 280 calories, and a can of soda is 150 calories a better alternative is a small to medium glass of fresh fruit, 1/2 cup of canned fruit or juice or 1/4 cup of dried fruit.

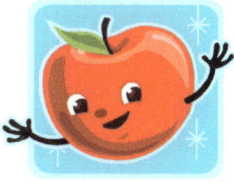

Head outdoors during your lunch break

Stepping outside can be the tonic you need.

Whether you can only take a 10-minute break or have the luxury of a longer lunchtime, heading outside to do some physical activity is a smart move during your workday.

Demanding workloads and looming deadlines make it difficult to stick to the best laid exercise plans. But if you're stressed, anxious, or just plain weary an exercise break serves as the perfect pick-me-up. Time and again research has shown that physical activity alleviates stress and depression, increases energy, and improves overall wellbeing.

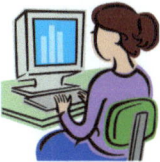

Aside from that simply getting a break from your computer or workstation is important for restoring some mental clarity.

Depending on how much time you have and the facilities available around you Workplace consider the following:

Ask a buddy to walk for 10 to 20 minutes with you, a brisk walk is ideal activity for working the muscles and joints without placing them under excessive pressure, it expands the lungs, improves metabolism, boots bone strength, tones the heart muscles and helps prevents the clogging of arteries. Don't be tempted to skip your walk if you can't find 20minutes as little as 10 minutes a day has been shown to bring health benefits such as helping to control weight and blood pressure.

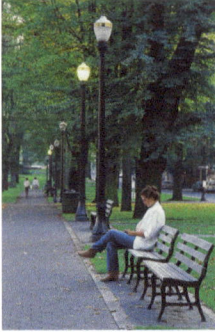

Head to the local park with the weather getting warmer consider swapping the indoors for some green space. Spending time with nature and getting away from your concrete jungle is known as a stress buster. Being outdoors in the daylight energies you.

You can use the local park for a leisurely walk, but if your preference is for a harder workout try some sit ups and press ups on the grass and use park benches for stretching, step ups and triceps dips.

If you like to sprint pick two trees about 30 meters apart and run from one to another then jog back.

Walk or jog up a hill, or a flight of steps. It's a cardiovascular workout that burns plenty of kilojoules and is excellent way to tone the legs and buttocks.

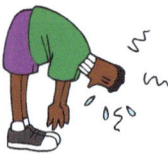

Remember to do light stretches before doing any jogging or running up stairs to help loosen up your muscles. Stretches should be held for no longer then 15-30 seconds but no matter how long you hold the position, you should never feel pain.

Stretch until you feel tension but if there's pain you have gone too far and need to back off, stretching is vital for good posture and helps imbalance in the body, as well as relieving muscular tension tightness and exercise soreness.

It can prevent injuries, improve physical performance, and reduces the risk of developing low back pain. Stretching boosts your energy and circulation and can help improve your sleep.

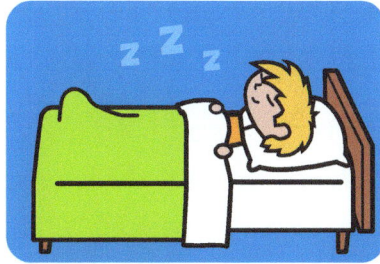

High Cholesterol and Your Health

High cholesterol is a big and invisible danger; many people tend to ignore the dangers associated with it because they can't really tell what's going on. Having high cholesterol can lead to serious health problems if left untreated.

It is important to do all that you can to keep your cholesterol levels at a healthy level and get your cholesterol checked regularly.

A cholesterol check involves a blood test which you need to fast 12 hours before having, this is the way your physician will test your cholesterol levels. Your HDL, LDL, and triglyceride level your HDL is referred to as "good cholesterol," as this form of cholesterol prevents artery blockages. Your LDL level is the one you should be concerned about, as this type of cholesterol is what builds up and creates blockages in your arteries.

While anyone can suffer from high cholesterol, ultimately a patient's background will be the deciding factor as to whether they will be at risk for more serious health complications. A patient with high blood pressure, smokes, is overweight or has a background that may lead to the possibility of heart trouble may increase the risk of heart problems due to high cholesterol. that is why this test is so important.

The blood test known as a lipid panel is sent to a lab and the results are given back to your physician who will then inform you of the results.

You will be advised of your LDL, HDL, triglycerides, and the total cholesterol levels. While the acceptable numbers for each vary by individual only your physician will be able to tell you what the appropriate levels should be and how your results compare. Your physician will then assist in lowering your cholesterol should it be high. If you find that you have been diagnosed with high cholesterol working with your doctor and make some significant changes to your lifestyle.

Stopping bad habits will assist in lowering high cholesterol. When paired with a diet that is cholesterol-friendly and proper exercise your health you will notice a great change. Don't let high cholesterol be a silent killer - *take steps to protect yourself.*

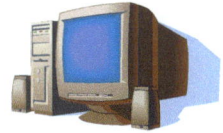

Don't be a norm get out and start exercising loose that weight and find the healthier new you.

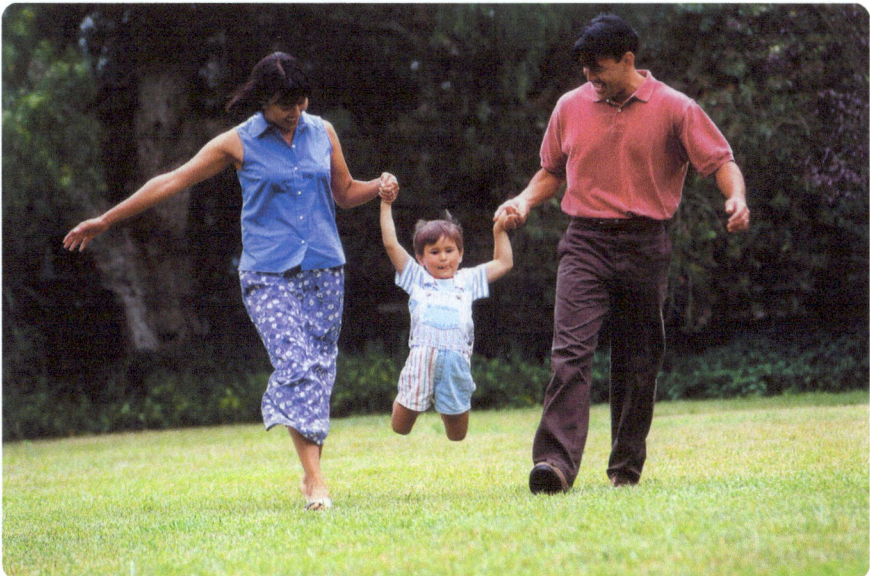

Fats and cholesterol

Cholesterol

Cholesterol is a fatty substance produced naturally by the body and found in our blood it has many good uses but can become a problem when there is too much in the blood.

There are two types of cholesterol - 'good' (HDL) cholesterol and 'BAD' (LDL) Cholesterol. LDL cholesterol is the type of cholesterol that clogs blood vessels and HDL helps unclog blood vessels.

If you have a high level of cholesterol, you can reduce it by changing your eating habits and have a healthier lifestyle.

Fats

Just like cholesterol, all fats are not bad. It is beneficial to have a certain level of fat. Fats in food are a mixture of saturated, mono-saturated and poly-saturated fats. These different types of fats have different effects on your cholesterol level.

Types of fats

Saturated fats

Saturated fat is found mainly in animal-derived food sources such as dairy products and meat. Two plant sources of saturated fat are coconut and palm oil and these are often used in processed foods such as biscuits, pastries, chips, butter, dairy foods, snacks and takeaway foods. Saturated fats tend to raise LDL cholesterol in the blood and can increase the risk of heart disease, obesity, diabetes, and certain cancers.

Polyunsaturated fats

Polyunsaturated fats help to lower blood cholesterol if your meals are low in saturated fats; examples of foods are fish, plain nuts, (walnuts, hazelnuts and Brazil nuts) and polyunsaturated margarines and oils. Polyunsaturated fats can be divided into omega-3 and omega-6 fatty acids.

Monounsaturated fats

Monounsaturated fats are found in vegetable oils (canola, olive, and sunola), some margarines, avocados, lean meats, chicken, eggs and fish, plain nuts (peanuts, cashews, and almonds). Monounsaturated fats can help lower blood cholesterol if your meals are low in saturated fat.

Fats

Fats are an essential part of our diet to provide energy and growth. Fats are the most concentrated source of energy available to our body; however, the average person eats far more fat than required for good health.

Many popular diets are difficult to adhere to and are not enjoyable. Eating should be pleasurable, and it is important to consume a wide variety of foods for enjoyment and nutritional adequacy.

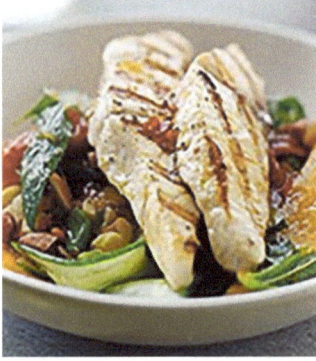

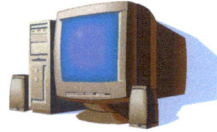

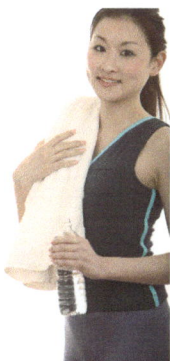

Water why is it important.

Do you drink enough water? You may think you are drinking enough, but many of us are unknowingly in a chronic state of dehydration. If you are not drinking enough, you may find that you are constantly tired and perhaps prone to headaches and generally feeling "FLAT". Our Bodies detoxification system is probably the most important component to optimum health and the one process that relies most heavily on an excess intake of clean water. We've all heard it said that we should drink a minimum of 8 glasses of water each day. Drinking the minimum will only help maintain a minimum level of health our bodies will use at least 8 glasses of water each day under normal relatively passive activity to maintain the basic bodily functions such as digestion, temperature control, joint lubrication and skin hydration. Each time we exhale blink our eyes or make any kind of movement we use up some of the available Water in our systems. Even the constant beating of our heart is a water consuming process. We're continuously depleting the available water level inside our body. In order for our body to properly perform the essential task of filtering and flushing out toxins we must consume a level of water above the minimum. The more of an excess that exists the more our body is able to rid itself of the elements that promote disease and aging. It's a beautifully simple process that can make a tremendous difference in the degree of health we achieve and maintain, but we must let it happen by consuming an abundance of clean, healthy water!

Our water quality is the only part of our environment that we can easily obtain total control over. With an abundant intake of clean healthy water we allow our body to perform all the healing processes it is naturally capable of in this age of fast food, synthetic medicines and complex lifestyles we tend to overlook the obvious. Our body is a water machine, performing millions of life-giving tasks with each passing second, and in each of these synchronized miracles there is one primary ingredient. The key is to drink regularly throughout the day, starting with breakfast. Keep a water bottle or jug nearby and aim to drink 1-2 glasses of water with every meal plus 1-2 glasses between meals.

Water is ideal, but other great fluids choices include green tea weak black tea (hold the sugar), herbal teas and low-fat milk. If you love your daily coffee don't despair caffeine in small amount is unlikely to do much harm, but if coffee and cola drinks make up many of your fluids for the day then you need to start visiting water cooler in preference to the coffee machine.

One can of soft drink contain about 10 teaspoons of sugar and sweetened juices are not much less.

Alcohol

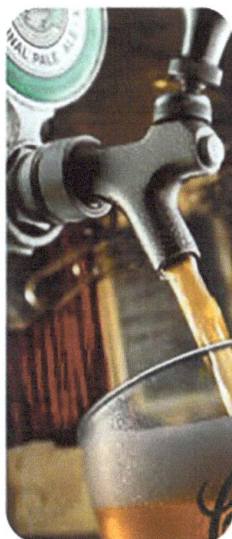

Negative effects of excess Alcohol Consumption.

Increased body fat levels Dehydrates and reduces *concentration, judgment and co-ordination and decreased* strength power and endurance.

Small amounts of alcohol consumed on a regular basis can have a positive effect on health.

As we get older however an excess of alcohol can lead to serious health problems.

Large volumes of alcohol may contribute to impaired liver function increased blood pressure, damage to brain cells and obesity. A number of studies have shown that a small and regular intake of alcohol may actually have positive effects on heart and health, however the mechanism is unclear.

Low to moderate alcohol intake is considered:

WOMEN — 2 standard drinks per day (on average)

MEN— 4 standard drinks per day (on average)

Plus two alcohol free days per week remember a 'Standard' drink may be far less than the volume you may normally consume.

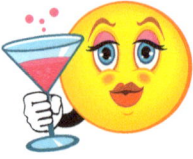

A standard drink of beer is 285ml.

It should be clear that there is no amount of alcohol that can be said to be standard for everybody,

These are general guidelines only.

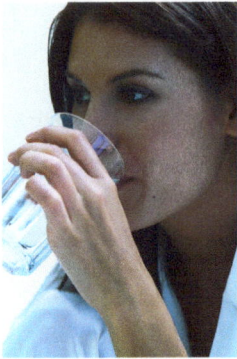

Choose water as your preferred drink.

Getting started

Although many people today need to lose weight there is still over one third who stays fit and healthy through regular exercise and healthy eating habits. If this sounds like you then it is important to choose a mix of foods that provide adequate fuel with enough nutrients to meet the demands of regular exercise. In today's environment we are busier than ever before and many of us are suffering from ongoing tiredness. The food and fluids you consume have a direct impact on your energy levels. Eating well will help you to feel fresh and alert everyday. Being healthy and active also enables you to cope with stress and may reduce the risk of depression.

3 Simple actions each day can help get you started.

DRINK PLENTY OF WATER

EAT 2 SERVINGS OF FRUIT

EAT 5 SERVINGS OF VEGETABLES

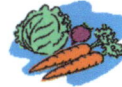

It sounds easy but putting it into practice can sometimes be a challenge.

By increasing your knowledge of different foods, their basic nutrient content and preparation techniques it is possible to eat tasty and healthy foods everyday.

So, Make Start Now

By making your health a priority, it becomes easier to introduce and maintain positive lifestyle change—there is nothing stopping you.

Why fad diets don't work

We all know that fad diets don't work, and eating whatever you like whenever you like doesn't work either. The key is to find something in between, a balance of healthy foods, while still including some of the foods you love to eat. The problem with diets is that they are restrictive and difficult to maintain. Add to this the likelihood of fatigue, due to low blood glucose levels, constipation, headaches, bad breath, and potential nutrient deficiencies and this all points towards the fact that diets are not a good idea. Cutting out food groups such as breads, cereals, fruit, and dairy foods can lead to inadequate intake of certain nutrients which can lead to fatigue and illness. Limited food choices can also lead to binges and can precipitate negative eating patterns. You can achieve major improvements in health and energy levels by changing your approach shopping, cooking and eating. Make your foods work for you, rather than against you!

THIS IS A FEW GUIDELINES

Enjoy a wide variety of nutritious foods	Take care to
Eat plenty of vegetables. and fruits	Limit saturated fat intake.
Eat plenty of breads, rice, pasta! cereals, noodles.	Choose foods low in salt.
Include lean meats, fish, Poultry.	Limit alcohol intake if you choose to drink.

Include milks, yoghurts, and cheeses.	Consume only moderate amounts of sugars and food containing added sugars.
Reduced fat varieties should be chosen where possible.	Prevent weight gain: Be physically active and eat according to your energy needs.
Drink plenty of water	Care for your food: prepare and store it safely

A nutritionally complete solution to weight control

A commonsense approach to nutrition includes low GI carbohydrates packed with soluble and insoluble fiber, low-fat sources of protein, and beneficial fats.

And by eating small low-calorie meals frequently throughout the day, you will create a calorie deficit without going hungry, making it easier for you to start controlling weight.

A better choice is to eat low GI foods which keep blood glucose levels more stable helping to reduce hunger cravings, leave you feeling satisfied longer, and controls *your appetite more easily.*

SOME MORE HELPFUL TIPS

- Clean all of the junk food out of your home & office!
- Avoid vending machine!
- Remind yourself that a NEW BEGINNING for you has started!
- Have a plan for dealing with tough times!
- Don't get too hungry have all of your meals and snacks
- REMEMBER look forward to eating the food you love in MODERATION!
- Always eat breakfast. People who skip breakfast end up eating more calories during the day.

☞ Don't eat after 8.30pm in the evening!

☞ Give yourself nonfood awards

☞ Remember that weight control can reduce the likelihood of developing high cholesterol.

OBESITY- related DISEASES

☞ Set goals & review them daily.

☞ Keep track of your progress.

☞ Ask for support.

☞ Use a buddy system.

☞ Plan.

☞ Always keep a diet bar with you for a healthy snack on the run.

☞ Avoid strenuous exercise Go slow!

☞ Try adding spices or flavorings to your shakes for variety.

☞ Blend shakes with ice for a thicker consistency.

Get moving any way you can!

While using any weight control method you should also walk up to thirty minutes a day, or about 3,000 steps. Buy yourself a pedometer to keep track of how many steps you take, gradually work up to 15,000 steps a day. Join a walking group or start one yourself start with a short 30 min walk or 3 x 10 minutes (if you are just starting out) walk on your lunch break.

Meet a friend for a walk and coffee. Make moderate, consistent exercise a part of your daily life, to control weight and to take advantage of the many health benefits that exercise can bring into your life.

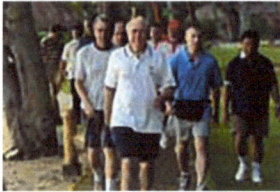

Repair the damage, lose the weight

Wind back the clock NOW!

Live longer, live healthier

Exercise burns calories it builds muscle mass which raises your metabolism and helps reduce stress and depression, which leads to overeating for many people.

Join a gym and have an exercise program tailored to your needs. Go jogging around the streets, parks or on the beach on the treadmill, swim, ride a bike or for something different take dancing lessons. Have a friendly tennis match, or go bush walking, play golf its unlimited what you can do. Turn off the TV and find time for a workout that will work with your schedule. Consider hiring a personal trainer and reward yourself for your progress.

Why do we put on Weight?

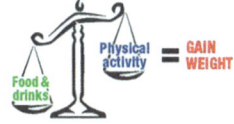

Body weight is affected by several factors.

- The amount of energy (kilojoules) that we put into our bodies from food and drinks.

- The amount of energy (kilojoules) that we use up through physical activity and other daily activities.

- Put simply, it's all about what goes in and what gets used up then you will gain weight.

- If you take in the same amount of energy (kilojoules) through food and drink that you are using through physical activity and daily activities, then your weight will stay the same.

- If the amount of energy (kilojoules) you take in through food and drink is less than what you are using through activity and daily activities, then you will lose weight.

Healthy weight loss takes time so don't be impatient Changes need to be for long term-make changes to your eating patterns and physical activity levels so you can live with the changes for the rest of your life. It's about you! Make changes that suit you, not what suits someone else. Take small steps and don't be put off by slow progress you may lose weight one week, and then go for a few weeks without losing any. Forget the scales your weight can go up and down from day to day. Weigh yourself once a week.

Measure your achievements in other ways rather then by how much you weight. For example: whether your clothes are looser, if you've cut down on TV. If you can do things without getting tired. Small amounts of weight loss or stopping weight gain will have a big impact on your overall health.

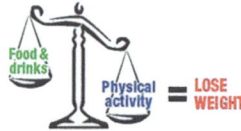

Seek advice and guidance first from your doctor, or an accredited practicing dietitian about your weight before starting any weight lose program.

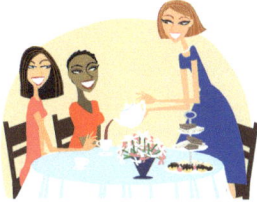

Don't Let Friends and Family Sabotage Your Diet

One of the biggest obstacles to any weight loss plan is getting around the many subtle and not so subtle ways that family and friends use to sabotage your diet.

While they are not even aware they are doing it, the tactics used by those closest to us have the potential to be the downfall of our most well-intentioned efforts to lose weight.

In some cases, family and friends feel insecure regarding your plans to lose weight and may begin practicing various tactics that are aimed at derailing your diet plans. They may complain about the amount of time that you spend working out; and deliberately schedule other activities that conflict with your scheduled exercise times. Shower you with tempting and fattening foods. Make pointed observations that you don't look as though you've lost weight or make predictions that you will gain all the weight you've lost.

Usually, this type of tactic stems from the fact that they are afraid your change in lifestyle may affect your relationship with them. This is especially true in relationships concerning husbands/wives and other romantic partners. There may be a very real concern present that you will notice others when you become slim.

In other cases, the tactics employed from those closest to you may not result from insecurities, but rather from a lack of knowledge. They simply may not recognize that offering one teensy slice of chocolate cake could set you back an entire week in your diet plans. Or perhaps they truly do not realize the health risks those extra pounds are presenting to you.

This type of behavior from those closest to us can be disheartening when we are already feeling vulnerable. Fortunately, there are several tactics you can use to withstand even the worst tactics friends and family may throw your way to sabotage your diet.

First, don't accuse friends / family of the tactics they are using. Instead, explain how much it means to you to lose weight and become healthier. Try to turn this into a way to spend more time together and bond by asking them to be your weight loss buddy.

Not only will this provide the back-up support you need, but it will help it will help to eliminate the feeling of insecurity they are experiencing as you begin to reveal the new you. When friends and family express judgmental feelings the first thing you should do is realize that these statements are more about their own feelings of inadequacies. Try not to take it personally. Instead, focus on the fact that you are doing something healthy for yourself. Be sure to let those closest to you know the guidelines for your diet. In some cases what appears to be sabotage could simply be the result of not having enough information. If you find certain areas are especially weak points for you, tell your family and friends in so that they can help you meet your weight loss goals.

A NEWER SLIMMER YOU

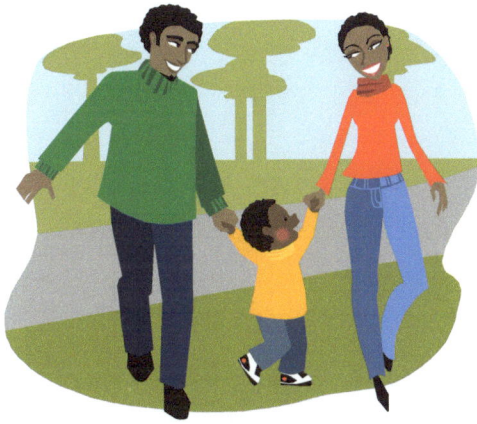

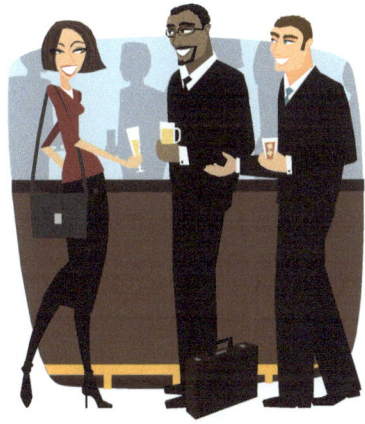

LOW GI
MEALS & SNACKS

Eating low GI foods throughout the day can help keep your blood glucose

levels stable while providing lasting energy. Here are tips to maintain a low G.I diet. Try these suggestions for breakfast, lunch & dinner.

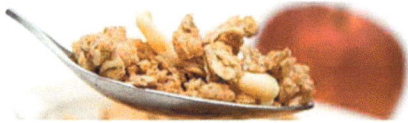

LOW GI BREAKFAST

A Nutria meal shake100% stone – ground, whole wheat toast topped with low sugar, natural peanut butter, and sliced banana.

Light yoghurt mixed with fresh fruit and muesli.

Rolled oats cooked in fat-free milk with dried apricots and nuts.

Sourdough French toast topped with natural apple sauce.

All-bran muffin with low-sugar and fruit topping fruit.

Buckwheat pancakes topped with fruit.

Multi-grain waffles topped with melted low-fat cheese; fruit Rye bread topped with light cream cheese fruit.

Vegetable omelets, extra lean turkey bacon, whole grain toast Low-fat cottage cheese with fresh fruit and almonds.

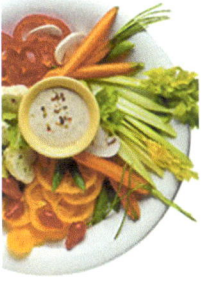

LOW GI LUNCHES

A light afternoon meal will help you get through the day. If you order out, substitute High GI sides such as chips- choose cottage cheese, vegetables, salads, whole-Grain breads, include low-fat protein.

Here are some other ideas for lunch:

- ☛ Homemade or canned soups, vegetable, lentil, black bean, split pea soup.

- ☛ Minestrone or barley (feel free to add extra vegetables).

- ☛ Sandwiches made with lean meats on whole grain.

- ☛ Pumper nickel or pita bread, fresh vegetables, fruit salad.

- ☛ Veggie burger with lettuce, tomato, onion and mustard on whole-wheat bun, cottage cheese.

- ☛ Pasta salad with vinaigrette dressing; assorted fresh vegetables and low- fat cheese.

- ☛ Mixed green salad with grilled chicken and vinaigrette dressing; whole wheat topped with natural peanut butter.

- ☛ Vegetable quiche, sliced tomatoes, Fruit.

- ☛ Light yoghurt with fruit, whole – grain muffin with melted low – fat cheese.

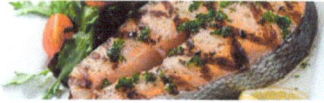

LOW GI DINNERS

Enjoy the many low GI possibilities available for dinner.

Watch out for hi-GI side's dishes and large portion sizes that could sideline your healthy habits.

Here are some tips to keep your dinner healthy.

1. Enjoy the many low GI possibilities available for dinner. Limit intake of HI GI starches - baked or instant mashed potatoes, fries, instant rice, stuffing mixes, refined white breads.

2. Choose low GI starches like pasta salad, wholegrain or sourdough breads, baked sweet potatoes, small new potatoes, corn, peas, or basmati rice.

3. Fill up on fresh, non-starchy vegetables and leafy green salads.

4. Include lean meats, such as chicken and fish, or substitute legumes for protein.

Try any of the breakfast or lunch suggestions for your evening meal.

LOW GI DESSERTS

You may not be able to have your cake and eat it too, but you can eat some tasty low GI treats. Try some of these sweets for dessert,

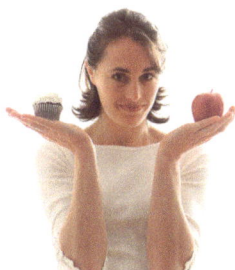

Sugar- free jelly or pudding layered with fruit.

Natural applesauce with light whipped topping

A small piece of Dark Chocolate or

A few chocolates covered strawberries.

Chocolate covered almonds or peanuts.

Low-fat milk with oatmeal cookies, poached fruit or baked apples with dried fruits and nuts.

LOW GI SNACKS

A NUTRITIONAL bar or FIBERGY bar is better for a snack then HI-GI foods.

Here are some tips.

1. Small handful of shelled nuts.

2. A bowl of low-fat popcorn,

3. A few wholewheat crackers topped with low-fat cheese.

4. Celery or banana topped with natural peanut butter.

5. Some whole-wheat pita chips topped with hummus.

6. A handful of baked tortilla chips with fresh salsa.

7. An apple or string of cheese.

8. Dried or Fresh fruit.

9. Hardboiled eggs.

10. Fresh cut vegetables.

11. Oat bran muffin.

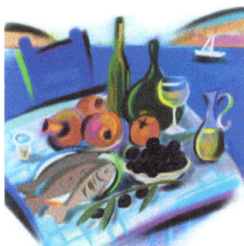

FOR MAINTIANING A LOW GI DIET WHEN EATING OUT.

Let's face it, everybody loves eating at a restaurant now and then, but it seems almost impossible to make good food choices when faced with so many options.

Here are some suggestions for eating well when you're eating out:

- Avoid buffets and other all-you-can-eat restaurants.
- Don't go when you're starving; eat small snack first.
- Limit alcoholic beverages.
- Keep your hands out of the bread basket.
- Go for the salad bar.
- Order items that have been prepared healthfully: steamed, broiled, roasted, etc.
- Don't be afraid to ask for substitutions.
- If portions are too large, split yours with someone.
- Keep low GI foods in mind and order the best choice available.

The following are some tips for specific types of restaurants:

CHINESE

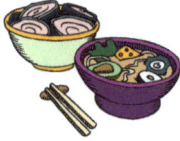

Order traditional dishes that feature moderate portions of proteins (meat, or tofu).

Stir-fried with assortment of vegetables and tasty sauces.

Avoid the fried foods and white sticky rice, order brown rice if available.

Broth-based soups like hot and sour, egg drop, or wonton are good choices.

Order foods cooked in black bean, oyster, Szechuan, or hot mustard sauce.

Chili sauce, Steamed dim Sims or spring rolls.

FRENCH

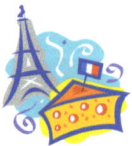

Look for Mediterranean-style items.

Avoid the bread and high fat sauces.

Order broiled, steamed, or poached foods.

Choose tomato/wine sauces, broth-based soup.

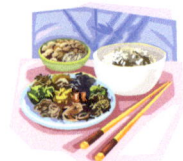

GREEK

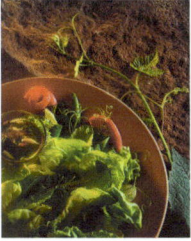

Choose roasted lamb or chicken dishes prepared with lemon and Yoghurt, order Greek salads.

Avoid the filo-dough, mounds of feta cheese and puddles of olive oil.

Try baked fish and chicken dishes that are healthy prepared.

INDIAN

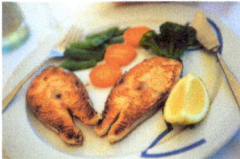

Order healthy prepared legumes, chicken, fish, and vegetables.

Choose basmati rice as a side in baryonic and chapatti bread.

Try the tomato-based sauces and Tandoori dishes and traditional Vindaloo.

ITALIAN

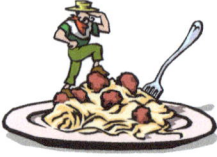

Steer clear of the white bread and creamy cheese sauces.

Choose tomato or Marsala sauces.

Order a half portion of pasta and combine it with a salad.

Go for the thin crust pizza loaded with vegetables and low-fat cheese.

JAPANESE

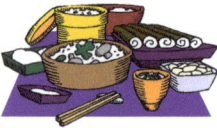

Try miso soup and soybeans for an appetizer.

Limit the sticky rice (ask if brown rice is available) and avoid tempura.

Choose sashimi, yakitori, sukiyaki, and grilled dishes.

Order udon or soba noodle.

MEXICAN

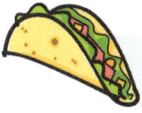

Stay away from the cheese and refried beans.

Order grilled seafood and chicken dishes, tacos, burritos, fajitas, enchiladas with beans.

Ask for low- fat cheese, wholewheat tortillas, and light sour cream.

Limit guacamole. And toppings such as salsa and mashed avocado.

THAI

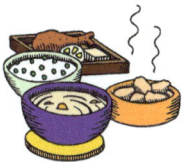

Order dishes that combine proteins (meat or tofu) with vegetables. Choose curry chilli, basil, lime, and fish sauces. Opt for long grain rice over white rice, soups and hot pots.

Rice paper rolls, fresh spring rolls and fish cakes, lean meat, or seafood skewers. Steamed rice or noodle dishes, stir fried or salads with seafood, vegetables or tofu with oyster sauce, garlic, ginger. Try Pad Thai and other stir-fried noodle dishes. Ask for less oil to be used in the preparation of these meals.

LEBANESE

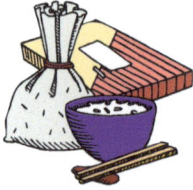

Lebanese bread with chickpea or eggplant dip, unless you can see excessive oil in the dips. Stuffed vegetables (Drain sauce), cabbage rolls, or Tabbouli BBQ Kofta, or lentils with rice.

Double Dutch?

Want to know what other food types to avoid when you eat out?

Include these synonyms for the term 'saturated fat' on your limited food list!

- Alfredo pasta sauce made with full-fat cream.
- Aioli traditional mayonnaise flavored with garlic.
- Au beurre (with butter) often with cheese added.
- Béchamel sauce made with butter, often with added cheese.
- Béarnaise sauce made with butter, egg yolks and herbs.
- Brioche rich bread made with eggs and butter.
- Carbonara pasta sauce made with eggs, cheese, and pancetta (or bacon).

☛ Confit meat or poultry cooked in and preserved with fat.

☛ Frito Misto battered and deep-fried meat, fish and vegetables pieces.

☛ Hollandaise sauce made with egg yolks and butter.

☛ Pate usually made with lots of butter.

☛ Tempura seafood or vegetables fried in butter.

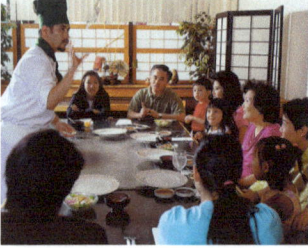

Be aware of smorgasbords.

They can encourage you to eat more then you need. Suggest sharing a dessert with someone at your table. Try to choose fruit-based desserts such as fresh, baked or canned fruit, or reduced fat custards, sorbets, or gelato.

Ask that no butter is added to vegetables.

Choose seafood dishes that aren't crumbed and fried.

Salad dressings and mayonnaise should be made from oils such as canola, sunflower, soybean, and olive oils. Ask for these on the side so you can add them yourself.

Choose a pasta dish with a vegetable-based sauce instead of a creamy one.

Beverages

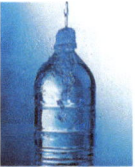

1. Choose water as your preferred drink.
2. Alcoholic drinks provide kilojoules but no important nutrients.
3. Keep your alcoholic drinks small and alternate with low kilojoules drinks like water, plain mineral water or diet drinks.

Fruit juices have the same kilojoules as regular beer.

If you are trying to reach a healthy weight drinking fruit juice instead of alcohol may not help you.

Take away foods!

Look for take-away foods that contain lean meats, lots of vegetables and cereals such as steamed rice, pasta and noodles.

Try to limit take-away foods such as pastries, pies, pizza, hamburgers and creamy dishes to once a week.

Below the good news is that there are healthier choices of take-away foods

Take away foods	Healthier choices
BBQ Chickens	Choose the breast meat. Remove the skin and fat and limit the gravy and stuffing. Serve with salad or vegetables rather than hot chips.
Italian	Choose pasta dishes with vegetable-based Sauces. Choose thin crust pizza with lots of vegetables. Try to avoid salami and sausage meats. Ask for lean meats and small amounts of cheese or reduced fat cheese
Asian meals	Choose steamed rice, mixed vegetables dishes, lean meats, (beef, lamb, pork or chicken), fish, and sea food and stir fries. Try to limit dishes based on fried noodles, battered, or crumbed deep fried meats or seafood, coconut cream/milk and ghee.

Hamburgers/ steak sandwiches	Ask for lean grilled meat and lots of salad. Where possible ask for extra salad and a wholegrain bun.

Lebanese/Greek	Choose donor/shish kebab/ souvlaki in pita bread with tabouli or Lebanese bread with salad.
Salad bars	Try to choose salads with dressing or mayonnaise made from oils such as canola, sunflower, soybean, and olive oils, or choose salads with dressing on the side.
Sandwiches and bread rolls	Ask for sandwiches and bread rolls to be made with margarine spreads and with reduced saturated fat fillings like lean meat, low or reduced fat cheese, skinless chicken, salmon, tuna, and plenty of salad vegetables.

Healthy breakfast tips and ideas.

Fast breakfast: simple ideas for people on the go.

- ☛ Keep a supply of wholegrain cereals and reduced-fat milk in the house.

- ☛ Prepare breakfast the night before by setting the table and getting things ready. Keep wholegrain cereal or wholegrain bread at work or take wholegrain snacks.

- ☛ Think of time saving items to keep in the kitchen bananas, reduced-fat yoghurt, small boxes of sultanas and cereal bars, or create a small snack pack of mixed dried fruit and some plain unsalted nuts.

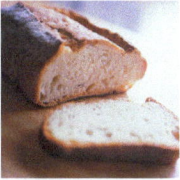

Bread, bread rolls and sticks.

Spicy fruit loaf spread with margarine.

Wholegrain bread rolls with reduced-fat cheese.

Half a wholegrain pita bread or flat bread spread with ricotta cheese or peanut butter and topped with apple or sultanas. Roll up and serve as a wrap.

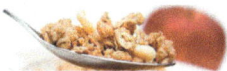

Cereal.

Split a dry breakfast wholegrain biscuit, spread with jam and topped with reduced-fat cheese.

Serve layered wholegrain cereal, reduced fat yoghurt and fresh fruit pieces in a disposable bowl or cup with a plastic spoon.

Serve wholegrain cereal with slices of fresh fruit such as bananas, apricots, peaches, strawberries or kiwi fruit. When using tinned fruit, use only those in natural juice or no added sugar.

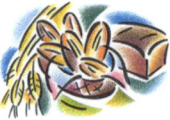

Wholegrain or Wholemeal, Crisp breads and rice cakes.

Add a healthy savory topping such as avocado and tomato or margarine and your favorite spread (E.g., jam or peanut butter). Spread with cottage or ricotta cheese mixed with walnuts and dates or sliced banana and cinnamon.

Top with a spread of margarine sliced tomato and pepper.

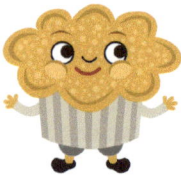

Wholemeal English muffins, Piklets and Scones.

Split muffin and spread with peanut butter or ricotta cheese.

Spread piklets or scones with margarine and top with ricotta and fresh fruit such as strawberry slices.

Top muffins with ricotta or cottage cheese and slices of fresh fruit.

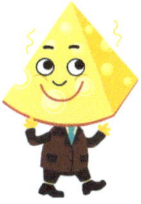

Meat and Cheese

Place a slice of reduced fat cheese or ricotta spread on wholemeal toast. Turkey stacks on a toothpick place a cube of lean turkey meat, a cube of reduced fat cheese and a cherry tomato, serve with a thick slice from a French stick.

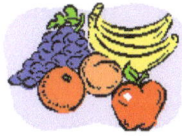

Fruit

Fresh fruit salad served in plastic cups and topped with reduced fat fruit yoghurt.

Cut oranges into four wedges and place in plastic bags.

Place sliced fruit onto wooden skewer freeze fruit into ice cubes. Serve frozen cubes in a plastic cup.

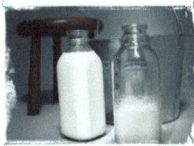

Milk.

Whip up a smoothie from reduced fat yoghurt, fresh fruit and a touch of cinnamon.

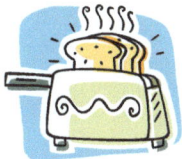

Toasty breakfast treats.

Toast wholegrain bread, wholegrain muffins or crumpets, spicy fruit loaf and then add delicious breakfast's toppings.

Spread with margarine and top it off with a sliced banana.

Toast spicy fruit loaf with margarine and then sprinkle with cinnamon.

Top your toasted base with a small tin of baked beans.

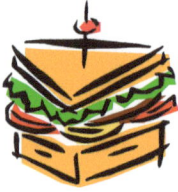

Using a Sandwich Maker to make toasted sandwiches of!

Toast spicy fruit loaf filled with banana and sultanas, apple, cinnamon and sultanas, or pineapple and banana.

Fresh reduced fat cheese and tomato or ham and tomato sandwiches. Use two slices of wholegrain or wholemeal bread and fill with baked beans.

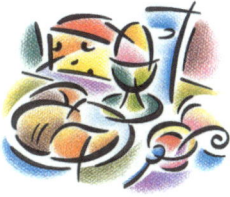

Hot breakfast hints

Try these great breakfast combinations!

- Toasted bread roll halved and topped with a mixture of chopped lean chicken or ham and tomato paste.

- Sprinkle lightly with a mixture of grated parmesan and reduced fat cheddar. Grill and serve warm.

- Mix a little mashed potato, cooked peas, reduced salt corn kernels, grated carrot and fresh pepper. Warm and serve in a cup with a spoon or on toast.

- Toast wholemeal crumpets and top with unsweetened tinned pineapple sprinkle with cinnamon and warm in pie oven cut into halves and serve.

- Breakfast pizza (serves 2) finely slice 1/4 green capsicum finely and 1 slice of fresh or unsweetened tinned pineapple into small pieces. Split 1 wholemeal muffin into two halves and spread tomato paste over each half. Place capsicum and pineapple on each, sprinkle with a pinch of oregano and top with reduced fat cheese slice on each half. Grill for 10 minutes until golden brown.

- If you like a hot breakfast other healthy ideas include baked beans, spaghetti, grilled tomato or braised mushrooms.

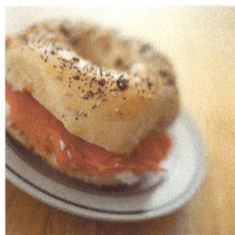

Fast, fresh recipe ideas

Skinny eggs and Ham on Bagels

Prep time: 20 minutes cooking time: 5 minutes

100g cherry tomatoes

125ml reduced fat evaporated milk

Fresh flat parsley leaves (12.)

Ground white pepper to taste.

Canola cooking spray

2 Whole meal bagels, halved.

4 eggs

100g shaved ham.

4 egg whites extra

Method

1. Cut the cherry tomatoes in half and place on a nonstick baking tray. Grill until soft and the skins begin to shrink. Remove and keep warm.

2. Put the parsley leaves on another baking tray, lightly spray with the oil and grill until crisp.

3. Put the egg, egg whites and evaporated milk in a bowl. Whisk to combine and season with a little white pepper.

4. Pour the egg mixture into a nonstick fry pan and cook over a low heat until the egg begins to set. Stir gently until just cooked. Do not over cook or the texture will not be smooth.

5. Toast bagels and top the bases with a little of the shaved ham, scrambled eggs, cherry tomatoes, and crisp parsley.

6. Serves 4

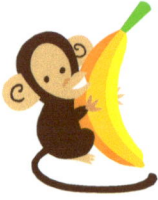

Crunchy Wrapped Banana

Prep time: 10 minutes cooking time: 5 minutes

4 sheets wholemeal lavish bread

1 teaspoon ground cinnamon

200g reduced fat ricotta

1 teaspoon caster sugar

2 tablespoons sunflower seeds

1 breakfast wheat biscuit, crushed.

2 tablespoons sultanas

4 bananas, halve and sliced /lengthways.

Method

1. Lay the lavish out flat on a clean surface.

2. Put the ricotta, sunflower seeds, sultanas, and wheat biscuit in a bowl and mix to combine.

3. Spread thick strips of the mixture along the centre of each lavish sheet.

4. Top with banana and sprinkle combine cinnamon & sugar mixture. Roll up put in a ridged sandwich press and toast until crisp and heated through.

   Serves 4

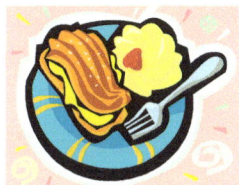

Avocado, spinach, Egg, and Tomato Wrap

Prep time: 10 minutes cooking time: 10 minutes

Canola cooking spray

50g baby spinach leaves, washed.

4 eggs

1 large avocado, sliced.

4 sheets wholemeal lavish bread

2 vine ripened tomatoes, sliced.

2 tablespoons reduced-fat cream cheese.

Cracked pepper to taste.

Method

1. Spray a nonstick fry pan lightly with canola spray. Heat the pan, add eggs and fry until just cooked. (Note eggs will cook further in the sandwich press).

2. While the eggs are cooking place the lavish on a clean surface. Divide the cream cheese among the four pieces and spread along the centre.

3. Top with spinach, avocado, tomato and egg and season with pepper

4. Roll up lavish bread & place in a ridged sandwich press and toast until crisp and heated through.

   Serves 4

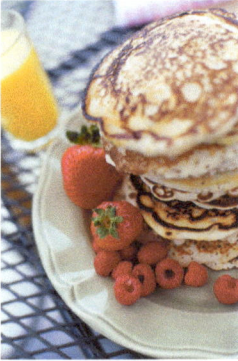

Jumbopancakeswithblackberryand honey

Prep time: 25 minutes cooking time 20 minutes

1 1/2 cup wholemeal self-rising flour

200g blackberries

1 teaspoon baking powder

40g low-fat margarine

2 tablespoons caster sugar

Canola cooking spray

1 egg, lightly beaten.

50g macadamia nuts, toasted.

2 egg white's

1/4 cup honey

375ml buttermilk

Method

1. Shift the flours and baking powder into a large bowl, stir in sugar. Make a well in the centre. Add combined egg, egg whites and buttermilk and whisk until the mixture forms a smooth batter. Cover and allow to stand, while preparing the butter.

2. To make the blackberry butter, put half the blackberries and the margarine in a bowl and mix

gently to combine, taking care not to puree the blackberries.

3. Heat a nonstick pan over medium heat and coat lightly with canola spray. Pour 1/4 cup of the batter into the pan and swirl gently to distribute the pancake mixture. Chop the nuts, put in a bowl, and stir with honey to combine.

4. Serve pancake stacks topped with a generous dollop of blackberry butter and a spoonful of macadamia nut honey. Sprinkle with the remaining blackberries.

Serves 4

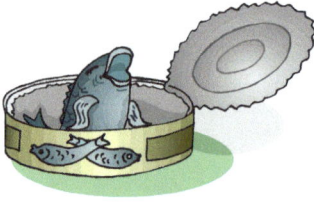

Tuna Patties.

Prep time: 10 minutes cooking time Potatoes: 15-18 minutes Patties: 5 minutes

500g Potatoes, peeled.

1/2 Onion chopped finely.

1/2 cup Parsley, chopped.

2 Eggs beaten.

Pinch coarsely ground black pepper.

2 tablespoons Canola or vegetable oil for cooking

Method

1. Cut the potatoes into 2-3 cm chunks.

2. Put into a large pot and almost cover with water cover and bring to boil then reduce to simmer until tender. (About 15 minutes).

3. Mean while prepare the other ingredients.

4. Mash potatoes and transfer the potatoes to a large bowl allow to cool.

5. Stir in remaining ingredients using both hands, form 1/4 cupfuls of the mixture into patties and arrange on a tray.

6. Heat 1 tablespoon of the oil in a fry pan and cook the patties until golden brown (about 2 minutes each side).

Serve these tasty patties on a bun with lettuce, tomato and mayonnaise or a wrap in fresh bread with tomato sauce. (Use a mayonnaise made from oils such as canola, sunflower, soybean, and olive oils).

Serves 4

Cranberry Rock Cakes Low- GI

1¼ cups self-raising flour

½ cup craisins (sweetened dried cranberries)

1 tablespoon raw sugar

200g tub low-fat berry yoghurt.

1x 56g egg, lightly beaten.

2 tablespoon vegetable oil

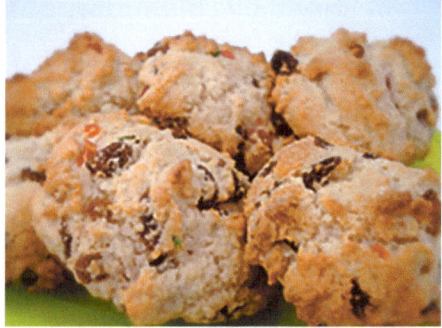

Method

1. Shift flour into large bowl, stir in craisins (cranberries) and raw sugar and make a well in the centre.

2. Add yoghurt, egg and oil and stir gently to form dough.

3. Drop tablespoons of mixture, about 4cm apart, onto a baking tray paper lined or greased, and flatten slightly.

4. Bake in oven preheated to 180c for 12-15 minutes or until rock cakes are lightly brown.

5. Cool on tray for 5 minutes, then transfer to wire rack to complete cooling.

Makes 12

These rock cakes will keep in an airtight container up to 3days.

Saver tips-- Low-GI Snacks

Foods with a low GI provide a **slow, steady release of glucose** into the blood stream.

Studies show a low- GI diet **reduces the risk of chronic disease** such as **TYPE 2 diabetes** and heart disease. Eating low-GI foods doesn't mean you have to spend a fortune on special diet foods. There are many **everyday foods** with low-GI to snack on:

- Baked beans
- Wholegrain bread and rolls
- Traditional porridge (not instant)
- Hommous dip with vegetable sticks
- Fruit loaf, fresh or toasted.
- Low- yoghurt
- Fresh fruit (pears, apples, and stone fruit)
- Dried apricots

Coping with Diabetes

Every day, in the United States and Australia more than 2000 new cases of diabetes are diagnosed. Type II diabetes, the most prevalent form of diabetes worldwide, often shows few or even no symptoms.

After eating, food is broken down into what is known as glucose, a sugar carried by the blood to cells throughout the body. Using a hormone known as insulin, that is produced in the pancreas which processes, the glucose into energy.

Because cells in the muscles, liver and fat do not use insulin properly in the body of a person with type II diabetes, they have problems converting food into energy. Eventually the pancreas cannot make enough insulin for the body's needs. The amount of glucose in the body increases and the cells are starved of energy.

This starvation of the cells, paired with the high blood glucose level can damage nerves and blood vessels. Leading to complications, such as kidney disease, nerve problems, and blindness and heart ailments.

There are many factors that can help to attribute to diabetes cases lifestyle, environment, heredity and those who are at risk should be screened regularly. Those that are already diagnosed with diabetes should aim to keep their glucose level under control.

But how do you know if you have type II diabetes? After all, it has few symptoms, often no symptoms in some patients.

However, if you notice an increased thirst or hunger, a change in weight, or blurred vision, getting tested for type II diabetes is necessary only your doctor will be able to help you find the treatment and steps necessary to be able to manage your life.

Simple changes such as eating right managing your weight and keeping your blood sugar level under control may be enough. However, you doctor may prescribe diabetes regulating medications to assist you in controlling your Type II diabetes.

Diabetes is a serious ailment with extreme consequences if it isn't treated properly. But if you follow your doctor's advice and maintain both your lifestyle and blood sugar levels, you can help to prevent the more serious consequences from occurring.

This article is for information purposes only and is not meant to treat, diagnose or prevent any ailment or disease. See your physician for proper diagnosis and treatment.

I CAN'T LOSS WEIGHT!

My weight has been up/down for as long as I can remember.

There are a few brief times in my life when I was able to force my weight under control through uncomfortable dieting and what felt like deprivation, and arduous exercise. None of it was easy and I couldn't maintain the loss for long and so the unwanted weight always came back.

I don't feel comfortable in my clothes and dread shopping for new ones. I stand in front of my closet looking for something to wear, and even though I have some nice things nothing appeals to me. I don't like the way I look no matter what I'm wearing. I know I'd feel so much better if I could lose some weight, but I feel powerless to do anything about my excess weight, so I'm very discouraged.

Sometimes this is hard for you to hear because you know from your personal experience in life that action does get results. You know that you have been able to shed unwanted weight by decreasing your food intake and there is no question in your mind that exercise helped. You may recall a successful experience where someone offered you an idea. Your enthusiasm could be attributed to your power of belief in the person who offered the idea to you, or it could be that the idea dovetailed precisely with beliefs of your own, but it's your enthusiasm we want to call your attention to.

The key to bringing your body to a new place is to see it differently from the way it is.

It is necessary to focus on the body that is coming and distract yourself from negative thoughts of your current body. Your choices right now do not include whether you are at your perfect body weight or not. You have no choice being at the body weight you are now; you will weigh about the same tomorrow as you do today, the next day and so on. Also, you are not, right now choosing between feeling fabulous or terrible.

You are not choosing between feeling enthusiasm or discouragement.

Your choices are more subtle and finer tuned than that.

You are making the simple choice of feeling a little better or a little worse.

You can choose to be happy or unhappy with yourself.

You can choose an unhappy thought or a happy thought. These are the only choices.

A short story

Imagine you are at a shopping centre, and you are moving in and out of many beautiful shops and there are hundreds of people moving in and out of them with you.

These individuals vary in size shape and wardrobe, but you predominantly notice the nicely dressed, nicely shaped, beautiful people all around you. As you see them you feel self-conscious. You turn and see your reflection in the window as you are walking and become aware of what you are wearing, and you are extremely unhappy about the way you look.

You feel agitated, discouraged, and unattractive, and now you are not enjoying your shopping outing at all. You have lost interest in the reason you came to the mall. You don't feel like shopping anymore. In fact, the only thing that appeals to you right now is the idea of getting something to eat.

The smell of food makes you realize you are hungry and that you need a snack. There are several choices within view and from the fragrances in the air you know there are more choices nearby. They all smell good to you, ice cream or candy or something more substantial like a sandwich sounds good. Actually, all of them sound pretty good to you right now your urge to find a quiet place to sit while you eat is becoming quite strong. You are trying to fight the urge to follow through on your impulse, it's much easier to just give in to it and get something to eat. As you wait in line at the ice-cream counter, you notice the slender people in line with you. They are annoying, and as you are annoyed, your urge for the ice-cream grows stronger still.

Before we offer guidance to assist you in improving your situation, we want to explain something that most people do not understand and, in fact have a hard time believing. Whether you gird up your willpower and walk out of the ice-cream shop or whether you go ahead and select and eat a tub of ice-cream. The action choice of one or the other makes no difference; it is what you are feeling that makes the difference, and how you are feeling about what you are doing.

In the beginning you may feel enthusiasm for some changes in your diet, and many would say, " Well, then, I don't see how this approach differs that much from just going on a diet as I've done so many times before." We ask you to be aware of how much easier it is this time in feeling enthusiasm rather than the discouragement that you have felt before.

You will also notice in this state of improved emotion you will find one appealing idea and then another. You will start rolling out a continuous path of good feelings and new ideas. You will begin to feel carried along by these new ideas rather than struggling to find them and before long you will begin to see physical results.

Upon seeing these results your feeling of enthusiasm will be even greater, then you are off and running toward the outcome that you have been seeking.

As you achieve your desired body weight (*and you will*) you will realise (*This time it wasn't difficult, and this time I'll keep it off*). I know what to do when I decide to do it to achieve whatever physical bodily condition I choose.

Consider this!

If being slender matches the emotion of happiness and you were to consistently eat ice-cream while feeling happy you would be a slender person who eats large quantities of ice-cream.

If your desire to be slender while you are currently not slender, matches the emotion of discourage you would be a fat person who eats ice-cream.

So in the beginning your thoughts may be something like this!

I am fat (unhappy)

I don't want to be fat (unhappy)

I'm so tired of being overweight (unhappy)

I don't like how I look (unhappy)

I don't like my clothes (unhappy)

I don't want to shop for clothes unhappy)

I've tried so many things (unhappy)

Nothing works for me (unhappy)

Remember, you do not have to fix everything just try to find a thought that feels good!

I wish I could find another way (happy)

My feet would feel better for sure (happy)

I like having choices (happy)

I like making deliberate choices (happy)

I like overseeing my actions (happy)

You're at work and have not been focused on your weight because you had things to accomplish. But now it is lunchtime and as you walk past the vending machine you feel an urge to buy a cookie. You put in your money the cookie drops and while you are unwrapping it the feeling of discomfort comes over you.

Here you go again you say, feeling the discomfort washing over you. But the urge is strong, and you take a bite of the cookie. You feel worse still as a strong feeling of disappointment comes over you.

But this time things are different from before because you have some positive momentum going from these statements you have been making about the subject of your weight. You remember, *it isn't about what I'm doing, It's about how I'm feeling while I'm doing it.* So, you pause and look at the cookie and you make the following statements:

I shouldn't be eating you (unhappy)

You'll only make me fatter (unhappy)

You are delicious, though (happy)

And you're not that big (happy)

I could eat some of you now and save some for later (happy)

I'm really making quite a big to-do overeating a little cookie (happy)

And sometimes I'll choose to eat you, and sometimes I'll pass (happy)

Right now, I'm going to eat you (happy)

And I'm going to enjoy you (happy)

You have just accomplished something that is rather unusual for you. You are eating the cookie and you have talked yourself into alignment and therefore still happy with your desire to be slender at the same time.

Don't look for immediate measurable physical results. Instead look for improvement in your mood, your attitude, and your emotions. When you're happy with yourself everything else will follow.

Abraham

MIND OVER MATTER

It may sound like a cliché but thinking yourself into shape really works.

Make a plan and have a vision!

Think about what you want to achieve perhaps you want to lose two dress sizes or be able to walk for 30 mins and increase your energy levels.

How will you achieve it? Hire a one-on-one trainer or talk a friend into walking with you?

And why you want it you refuse to buy new clothes in size 16 or 20 and climbing the stairs wears you out, and you feel tired all the time.

Commit your plan to paper and constantly envisage your *GOAL PHYSQUE.*

Make a firm decision!

Now that you know what you want, how badly do you want it?

Are you ready to give it your all? Sit down and write a promise to yourself that you will give 110 per cent and not make excuses and not give up.

You must be prepared to make sacrifices for the first 12 weeks.

Nothing worth changing is ever easy, instead of trying to fit your diet around your work commitments, family and social outings make the transformation process your priority. With the right attitude the 12 weeks will pass quickly so make sacrifices for this short time and you'll be amazed at what can be achieved. If your approach is half-hearted, you can't expect brilliant results.

Become selfish!

To achieve an amazing transformation, it has to be all about you. If you choose not to go to the pub for Friday night drinks, your friends will get over it. If friends or family have been holding you back or getting in the way of your goals, it's time to get selfish put yourself first. If you don't, you'll continually be disappointed with your results.

Alcohol for 12 weeks, forget that pizza, McDonalds, fried chicken.

Pull all thoughts of non authorised foods out of your head. Don't waste time wanting, looking at, or thinking about food that is not part of your plan. Think about what you can have, not what you can't have. Have plenty of water instead.

NO EXCUSES

There are no valid excuses if you want amazing results in 12 weeks. There are always alternatives, pay close attention to planning. Have contingency plans for emergencies. If you start making excuses, then you haven't made a total commitment then you are wasting your time. Make total commitment to do this. **<u>NO EXCUSES EVER.</u>**

I hope you enjoy reading this book and get some benefits from it as I have putting this together for you.

Ki9ds Health and how to get them Active.

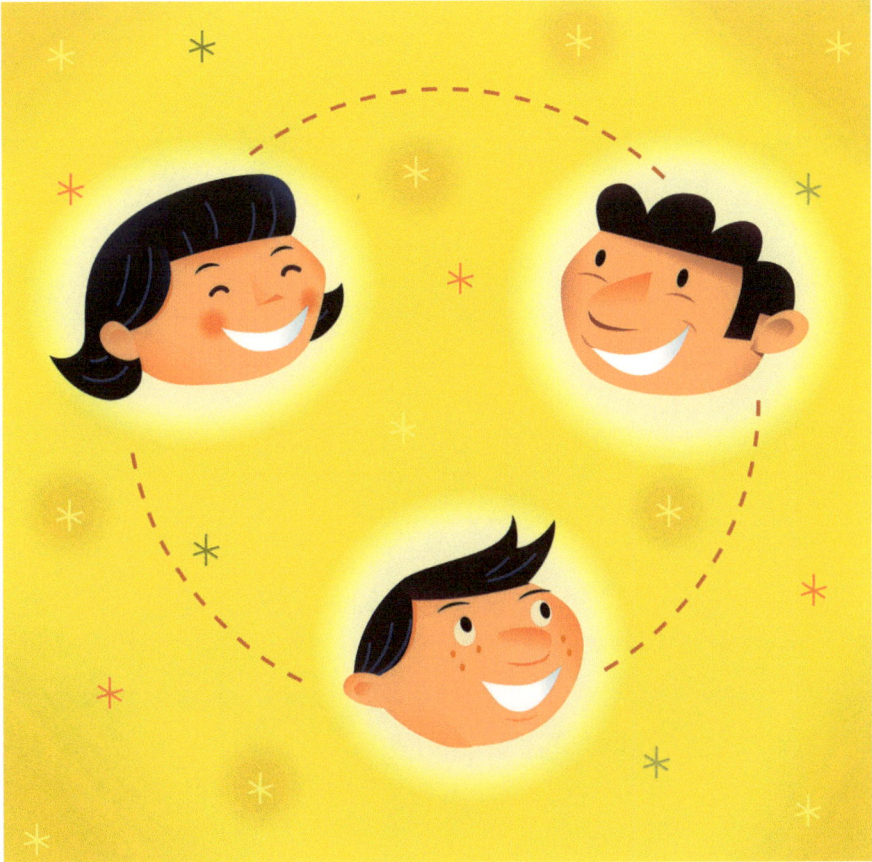

Contents

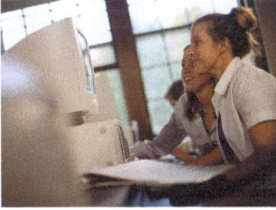

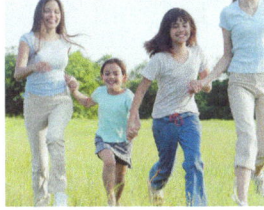

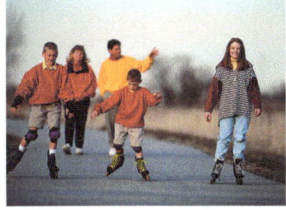

GET OUT! GET ACTIVE! GET HEALTHY!

This booklet covers nutrition tips for healthy eating and delicious recipes in the hope you get enjoyment using this handy guide.

Kids and Their Health - So much to do so little time! As every parent knows, 'today's kids have never been busier. More homework, and the fast pace of activities after school, and at weekend leaves less time for the fun of creating their own games and entertainment.

And if you think kids don't have enough time to relax, spare a thought for the parents who have the job of ferrying them around and doing their best for what is surely the world's hardest job.

It seems parents are spending much of their leisure time with their kids, but despite the demands, the world's toughest job is also a great joy. We love seeing our kids grow, learn, and develop. And more than anything our kids want to spend time with us.

So here's a guide to helping you get the most out of your time together.

Whether it's taking the ball out to the yard or going for a walk to the park or getting together with friends at the beach, the secret is in taking the first step and being active together.

If you resolve to do one thing differently for your kids, this year get them out of passive indoor play and into action in the great outdoors?

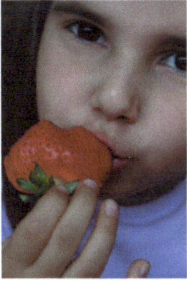

Healthy eating for active kids

Healthy eating gives kids the energy they need for their busy days. Here are some. great ways to make to make it easier.

MAKE BREAKFAST

The most important meal of the day it can be up to 12 hours since their last meal, so kids need to refuel for the day ahead. Give them healthy choices like cereal and milk, toast, English muffins, fresh fruit, eggs on toast, juice, and yogurt.

WATER WORKS

Get into the habit of taking water with them everywhere to keep them hydrated throughout the day.

SNACK SMART

Encourage your kids to take control of their health early in life by planning their own healthy snacks. This will help them look for a healthy diet as they grow older.

GET COOKING

Food is not just about good nutrition it's one of life's great pleasures. Encourage your children to help in the kitchen even young children can help peel carrots, pod peas, grate cheese, put together tacos or design their own healthy pizza topping. If they've helped, they will be more likely to enjoy eating it.

EAT AT THE TABLE

Avoid letting kids eat in front of the TV or the computer; get them into the habit of eating or snacking at the table or kitchen bench.

SLOW AND STEADY

Encourage them to eat slowly! This prevents overeating and aids digestion.

GET A BALANCE

Variety and balance is the key to helping your child enjoy a healthy diet. Aim to eat a variety of foods each day. Include fruit (2 serves) vegetables (5 serves) breads and cereals (5-6 serves) lean meat or fish (1-2 serves) and dairy products (3-4 serves). Children and adults need a variety of nutrients to help function and grow normally. By including a healthy variety of foods in our diet we can still enjoy the occasional treat.

TASTY EXPLORATION

Encourage your child to try different foods from different cultures. Exposure to lots of different tastes and flavors adds excitement to meals.

10 ways kids can get active.

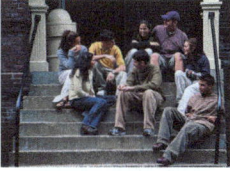

Whether it's playing with friends or family. Taking part in sports or joining regular family activities. Being active is good for everyone!

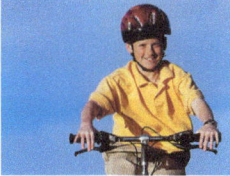

Get active. Early, active kids are more likely to become active adults so teach them to enjoy it now.

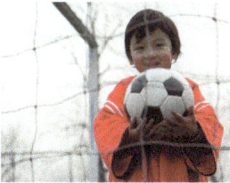

Variety! Variety, encourage kids to try a range of sports and activities to develop a range of skills and find one or two that they really like.

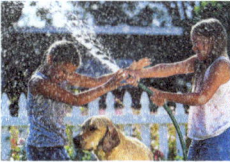

Have fun sounds simple but the basic rule is that sport and activity should be enjoyable.

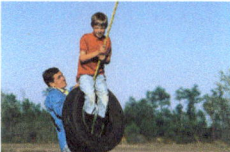

Take the lead because kids take their cues from parents, so make activity a regular part of your family routine.

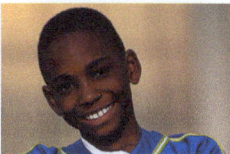

Give the toys a miss. Help kids get active by giving sporting rather than toys as gifts.

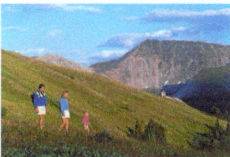

Try something new; develop a new family activity such as in climbing, bike riding, skiing, or sailing.

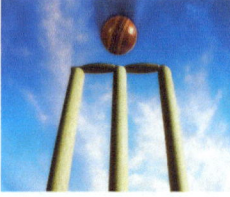

For an easy 20minutes of fun keep handy action toys such as touch football, basketball, or cricket, tennis ball in a spot easy to grab on the way out.

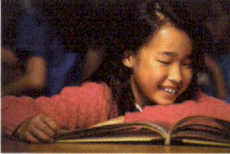

Find a balance help your child find their own balance of friends, physical activities, indoor play, and homework with unstructured play such as daydreaming, creating, thinking and reading.

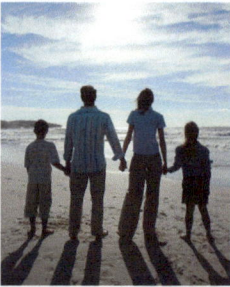

Give the chauffeur the day off 'that's you! Introduce children to the way we all once got around walking, riding bikes, or walks on the beach with them.

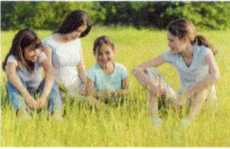

Every day aim for 30 /60 minutes of moderate activity, plus 20/30 minutes of stronger activity up to three times a week.

Children and Body Weight

Children who are active and enjoy healthy eating will usually have a healthy bodyweight. Poor health is associated with being very underweight or very overweight.

What if children are underweight?

Children who are underweight need to be encouraged to eat.

a variety of foods frequently throughout the day, and to stop.

play and other activities for these snacks.

What if children are overweight?

Children who are overweight should not be put on "diets." They need to be encouraged to be more physically active to limit their intake of 'HIGH-ENGERGY' snacks such as chocolate, potato chips, deep fried foods, confectionery& soft drinks. Overweight children also benefit from being encouraged to eat a wide variety of foods, for example, vegetable and fruits.

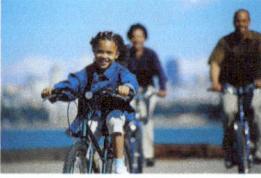

Family activities

Such as bike riding or visiting the playground, are great way to help children increase their physical activity and provide support for the child to manage their weight. If a child does appear to be overweight, it's important that they are not singled out as being different to other children. Being treated this way may itself cause low self-esteem and lack of confidence. Management of the child who is overweight requires help from a professional such as an Accredited Practicing Dietitian (APD) or Pediatrician. Food intake should never be restricted as inadequate food can lead to poor physical and mental development. As far as possible, the emphasis is on maintaining than losing weight and allowing the child to 'grow' into their weight.

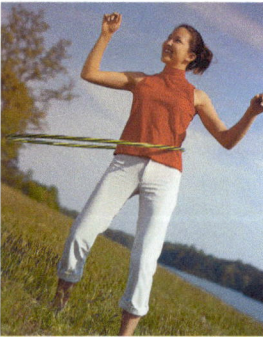

Body Image

The way an individual perceives his or her body, is called their body image. Unfortunately, society imposes particular body shapes and sizes as the 'ideal' for males and females; this influences our perceptions of our bodies and our value as a person. Children are also influenced by this concept of the ideal body.

Body shape is inherited, and no amount of physical activity and dieting will change it.

The way children perceive their bodies can affect their food intake, the way they perceive their abilities and hence their health.

It's important for children to understand their own body and learn that the physical changes that occur is part of growing up. The aim is to develop normal eating habits. Feel relaxed and comfortable with food, and not feel guilty or afraid to eat for fear of putting on weight.

Tips for helping your child have a healthy body weight and a healthy body image.

Encourage your children to enjoy healthy eating and to be physically active. Help children to understand that food is important for good health and teach them how to make healthy choices.

Be positive role models for healthy eating and physical activity. Have plenty of healthy food choices available and participate in the fun activity as a family.

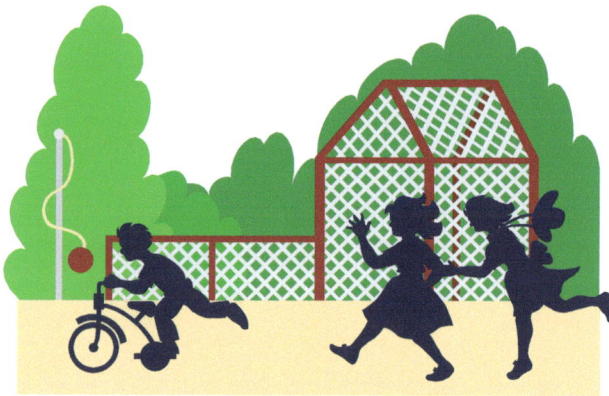

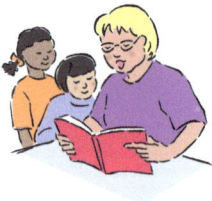 Encourage your children to develop a positive self-esteem and body image by helping them to understand there is no ideal body shape and that good health can be achieved by many shapes and sizes.

Make children feel special about them self and who they are. Help them understand that their appearance and body shape does not determine their value as a person.

Try to avoid making comments about body weight in general. Focus more on growth and less on scales. Weighing children who are already conscious of their weight can make them feel more uncomfortable.

Focus on improved fitness, health and having fun rather than on weight and food restriction.

Don't force children to 'exercise' or participate in activities that they do not enjoy-this can result in a negative attitude to physical activity throughout life.

If you think your child has a weight problem

Seek professional advice.

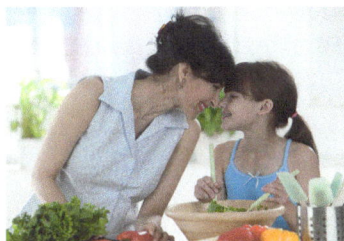

Snacks, Breakfast and Drinks for Children

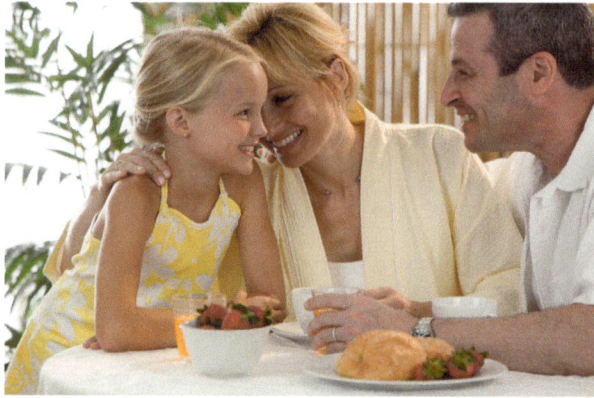

Snacks: an important part of children's daily food intake

Healthy snacks throughout the day are an important part of a child's daily intake. Children need to eat every few hours to keep up their energy levels and to ensure they have adequate nutrients. Of concern is the type of food they eat rather than how many times they eat food.

Often the types of foods chosen as snacks are low in dietary fibre and nutrients, and high in saturated fat and salt. Common examples are potato crisps and chocolate bars. Eating these foods occasionally is harmless. It's the frequent consumption that is a problem.

The easiest way to make sure that children choose healthier snacks is to provide them with plenty of choice. Offer a range of snacks options of varying colors, textures and flavors and try not to have less healthy snacks available in the home.

When preparing snacks for children, ensure you:

- ☛ Choose plant-based foods, for example fruit, bread, vegetables.

- ☛ Encourage children to understand a treat is an occasional, rather! than an everyday item.

- ☛ Make water a regular drink, with soft drink or juice as an occasional option.

Keep in mind that taste and interest are important factors in encouraging children to eat healthy snacks.

Examples of healthy snacks include:

- ☛ Fresh fruit, fruit kebabs, canned fruit in natural juice, cooked fruit.

- ☛ Vegetables stick with reduced-fat dips, plain corn on the cob.

- ☛ Homemade soup.

- ☛ Reduced-fat yoghurt (natural or fruit).

- ☛ Scones, pancakes or piklets, prepared with reduced-fat milk and margarine spread.

- ☛ Bread, crumpets, English muffins, rice cakes, crisp breads, or sandwiches.

- ☛ Unsalted nuts (not suitable for children under five); Dry biscuits with salad vegetables (for example tomato), reduced –fat cheese or dips.

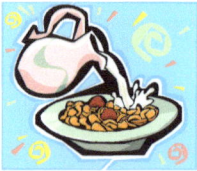

Breakfast

Breakfast provides energy to get us through the day as well as essential vitamins and minerals. Eating breakfast can improve memory and problem-solving skills and improve creative thinking and concentration. With a healthy breakfast children have the energy to play, be alert, concentrate in class and feel good about them self.

A healthy diet can include almost any type of food – breads, cereals and grains, fruit, vegetables, reduced-fat dairy products and lean meats. What people eat at breakfast time depends on a few factors including cultural background, religious beliefs, food preferences, and food time available.

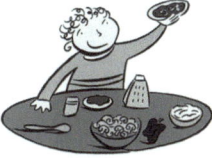

Examplesofahealthybreakfastinclude:

Toast or bread, with polyunsaturated or monounsaturated margarine spread plus a topping, such as jam, tomato, reduced-fat cheese unsalted peanut butter or reduced salt baked beans.

Rice or noodles on their own or with lean meat or vegetables; reduced-fat yoghurt, fruit, bread.

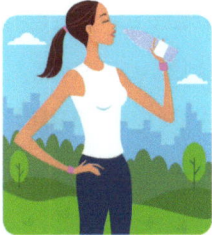

Drinks

It's a good idea to have a drink with breakfast.

Suitable drinks include water, reduced fat milk or tea.

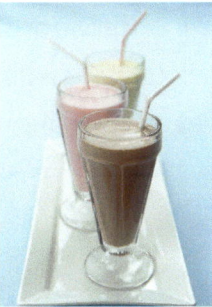

For those who don't have much of an appetite in the mornings, offer a smoothie as an alternative to a 'solid' breakfast. Combine reduced fat yoghurt, fresh fruit, some honey, and a handful of wheat germ.

It doesn't really matter how old you are water is essential for life!

Water is the preferred drink for children. While milk is important for adequate calcium intake too much can lead to poor appetite.

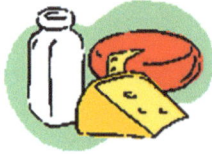

Three serves of dairy products daily.

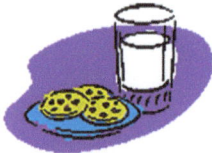

Including a glass of milk is recommended.

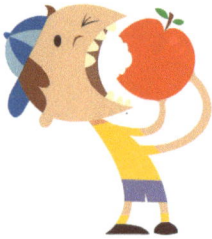

Children should be encouraged to eat whole fruit rather than drink fruit juices, and juices should be limited to one small glass per day.

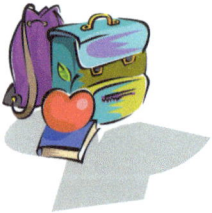

Good eating habits begin in childhood. For children to keep up their energy levels and get through a hectic day at school they need to eat a variety of foods.

This page provides simple, tasty and nutritious ideas to include in your child's school lunch box. The lunch box ideas below consist of a snack, lunch, and drink combination. Use the ideas provided in this page or make up your own. Try to include fruit and reduced fat milk, or another reduced fat dairy product in the lunch box every day.

Snack - Piklets with margarine and jam.

Lunch - Reduced fat cheese and chutney sandwich, with fruit in season and water.

Snack - Half a corn on the cob (pre-cooked and wrapped).

Lunch – Ham, mustard, and tomato sandwich with fruit in season and water.

Snack - Small tub reduced fat yoghurt (plain or fru

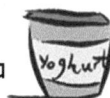

Lunch - Tuna, lettuce, and avocado in a wholegrain roll with fruit in season and water.

Snack - Small can or tub of fruit.

Lunch – Chicken and lettuce rolled up in Lebanese bread with fruit in season and plain reduced fat milk in a thermos (to keep it cold).

Snack - Veggie sticks (e.g., carrot, capsicum) with a small tub of salsa dip.

Lunch- Peanut butter sandwich with fruit in season a small tub reduced fat yoghurt (plain or fruit) and water. **(Please be aware of schools that call for peanut butter bans due to children that have an allergy to peanut butter).**

Snack – Fruit loaf with margarine spread.

Lunch – Rye bread sandwich using lean meats (choose sandwich meats) with small tub of carrot sticks, celery sticks, and cherry tomatoes and water.

Snack – Plain fruit-based muesli bars.

Lunch – Home made pizza (make your own pizzas the night before with Lebanese bread, tomato paste, veggies, and reduced cheese. They taste great cold the next day)! fruit in season and water.

Snack – Plain or fruit scone with margarine spread and jam.

Lunch – Egg and lettuce sandwich with fruit in season and water.

Snack – Banana, ricotta and sultanas wrapped in wholemeal lavish bread.

Lunch – Kidney beans (mashed), tomato, spinach leaves and avocado in a wholegrain bun with fruit in season and water.

Snack – Reduced fat cheese stick or triangle and sultanas.

Lunch – Chicken or turkey, celery, and lettuce sandwich with fruit in season and water.

Snack – Small tub of yoghurt (plain or fruit).

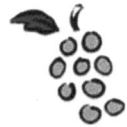

Lunch – Vegetable soup in a thermos served with a bread roll spread using margarine with fruit in season and water.

Nutrition tips

1. Children eat different amounts of food according to their growth patterns. For smaller appetites pack smaller serves cut sandwiches into quarters and cut up fruit into bite-size pieces.

2. Calcium is lacking in many children's diets provide a calcium-rich food like milk, cheese or yoghurt every day. Children under two years of age need full-cream milk and dairy products for extra energy. After two years of age gradually introduce reduced fat milk and dairy products.

3. Fruit has more fibre and less kilojoules than fruit juice. Make fruit a regular lunch box item.

4. Include water or fat reduced milk as a daily drink with fruit juice as an occasional treat.

5. Use margarine spreads or mayonnaise made from oils such as canola, sunflower, soybean, and olive oils.

Practical tips

1. Freeze drinks in the summer and use as the lunch box cooler (place inside box or strap it to the lunch box with an elastic band). This will help keep food cool as well as safe to eat.

2. Involve your child in choosing their own lunch from the range of healthy options provided in this book. It's okay if they eat the same food every day as long as their food choices are mostly healthy.

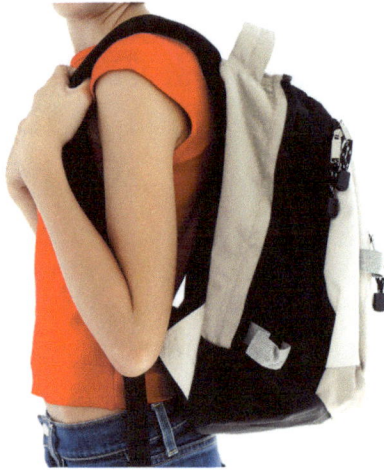

Some kids still need high GI foods for their active bodies to maintain their energy. But be careful not to allow your child to have too much high G.I foods. That will cause any weight problems later!

Sports Drinks

Nowadays there are so many sports drinks to choose from. Originally, these drinks were designed to bring out the best in elite and professional athletes. However, it is the length and your nutritional needs, not your expertise at doing it. Even recreational athletes can benefit from good use of a sports drink.

Sports drinks are designed for two main purpose to *replace fluids* lost during exercise and to *improve performance* by providing the muscles with fuel, please be careful of how many sports drinks your kids drink during their sports games they should only have one and maybe two for older kids.

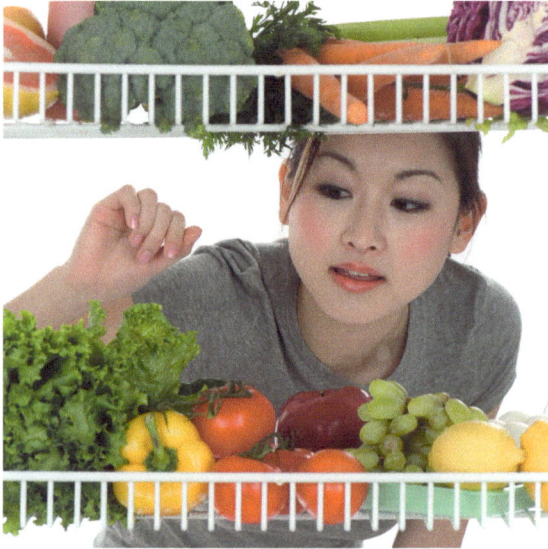

A HEALTHLY LIFESTYLE

LMDInvestments

2 Creese street Beaconsfield Qld 4740

Sydney Australia

Lorraineday@outlook.com

www.ingramcontent.com/pod-product-compliance
Lightning Source LLC
Chambersburg PA
CBHW040936030426
42335CB00001B/13